Fertile Feasts: 10 Power-Packed Recipes to Boost Fertility

Cooking Your Way to Fertility Bliss

Priscilla J. Schulz

Table of Contents

Overview

Welcome to "Fertile Feasts: 10 Power-Packed Recipes to Boost Fertility." In this book, we embark on a flavorful journey that intertwines the art of cooking with the science of fertility enhancement. The profound impact of nutrition on our overall well-being has been well-documented, and its influence on fertility is no exception. Understanding this connection forms the cornerstone of our exploration.

Within these pages, you'll discover an assortment of recipes meticulously crafted to harness the potential of nutrient-rich ingredients known for their ability to support fertility. Each dish is not just a culinary delight but a deliberate composition, aimed at nourishing the body and fostering an environment conducive to fertility enhancement.

Whether you're starting on this journey toward parenthood or seeking to optimize your health and fertility, these recipes are designed to empower and inspire. Join me as we delve into the realm of fertility-boosting foods, savoring the delightful flavors while embracing the potential they hold for a brighter, fertility-focused future.

Understanding the Connection between Nutrition and Fertility

The relationship between nutrition and fertility is multifaceted, impacting various aspects of reproductive health for both men and women.

For women, a well-rounded diet supports hormonal balance, menstrual regularity, and optimal ovulation. Essential nutrients like folate, found in leafy greens and legumes, are crucial even before conception as they reduce the risk of neural tube defects in the fetus. Iron-rich foods such as red meat, beans, and spinach are important to prevent anemia, which can affect fertility by disrupting ovulation.

Omega-3 fatty acids, commonly found in fish like salmon, support reproductive health by aiding in hormone regulation and improving blood flow to the reproductive organs. Antioxidants like vitamin C (in citrus fruits) and vitamin E (in nuts and seeds) help combat oxidative stress, which can negatively impact egg quality.

Conversely, diets high in processed foods, sugar, and unhealthy fats can lead to inflammation, insulin resistance, and hormonal imbalances, potentially affecting fertility. Excessive caffeine intake has also been linked to fertility issues, as it may interfere with conception by affecting ovulation and increasing the risk of miscarriage.

In men, nutrition significantly influences sperm quality. Zinc, found in foods like oysters, beef, and pumpkin seeds, is essential for testosterone production and sperm health. Vitamin C, abundant in fruits like oranges and strawberries, protects sperm from oxidative damage, enhancing their motility. Selenium, present in Brazil nuts and seafood, also supports healthy sperm production.

Conversely, diets high in saturated fats, processed meats, and excessive alcohol can impair sperm production and function. Heat from hot tubs or excessive saunas, combined with poor nutrition, can further impact sperm quality.

Maintaining a healthy weight is crucial for fertility in both genders. Obesity can disrupt hormone levels, leading to irregular ovulation in women and lower testosterone levels in men. On the other hand, being underweight can affect hormone production, potentially leading to irregular menstrual cycles and reduced sperm quality.

Ultimately, understanding the intricate link between nutrition and fertility underscores the importance of adopting a balanced diet rich in whole foods, vitamins, and minerals for couples aiming to conceive. Consulting with healthcare providers or fertility specialists can provide personalized guidance to optimize nutrition and maximize the chances of successful conception.

CHAPTER 1

SEEDS OF LIFE

1.1 Recipe 1: Super Seed Breakfast Bowl

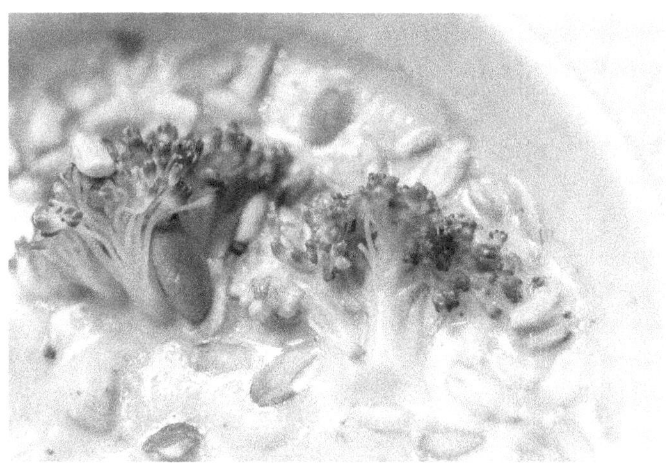

Start your day off right with this colorful breakfast dish, which is full of fruits and seeds that are high in nutrients and promote fertility. Hemp, flax, and chia seeds all work well as a great supply of omega-3 fatty acids, which are vital for healthy reproduction. Antioxidants and vitamin C, which shield cells from harm and support hormone regulation, are added by pomegranates and berries. Savor this filling and tasty breakfast bowl to start your day off well.

Ingredients:

- ¼ cup pomegranate arils

- ½ cup mixed berries (strawberries, blueberries, and raspberries)

- ¼ cup plain Greek yogurt

- 1 tablespoon each of chia, flax, and hemp seeds

- ½ cup almond milk

- 1 tablespoon honey

- ¼ teaspoon vanilla extract

Guidelines:

- 300 In a bowl, combine the mixed berries, pomegranate arils, Greek yogurt, chia seeds, flax seeds, hemp seeds, almond milk, honey, and vanilla essence.

- Give everything a good stir to ensure even coating.

- To achieve a thicker consistency, cover the bowl and refrigerate for at least 30 minutes or overnight.

- Garnish with more berries, pomegranate seeds, or honey drizzle, if you'd like, just before serving.

Tips:

- You can add agave nectar or maple syrup for a sweeter breakfast bowl.

- Top with a sprinkle of granola or chopped nuts for added crunch.

- Add a dollop of nut butter for extra protein and healthy fats.

- Layer the ingredients in a jar or other container to enjoy this breakfast dish on the road.

Benefits:

- Nourishes your body with essential nutrients

- Promotes overall well-being and reproductive health

- Supports fertility with omega-3 fatty acids, antioxidants, and vitamin C

- Provides a boost of energy and fiber to start your day

As part of a nutritious and well-balanced diet, savor our Super Seed Breakfast Bowl to help your fertility journey.

Additional Recipes:

- Smoothie for Fertility:
    - 1 cup mixed berries,
    - ½ banana
    - 1 cup spinach
    - ¼ cup Greek yogurt
    - 1 tablespoon almond milk
    - 1 tablespoon chia seeds should all be blended together.

- Poached eggs on avocado toast:

- Toast a piece of whole-grain bread, then place two poached eggs on top along with some avocado slices. Drizzle with balsamic vinegar and olive oil.

- **Nuts and Berries with Muesli:**
  - Cook half a cup of steel-cut oats in milk or water. Add some chopped nuts, mixed berries, and a honey drizzle on top.

1.2 Recipes 2: Quinoa-Stuffed Bell Peppers

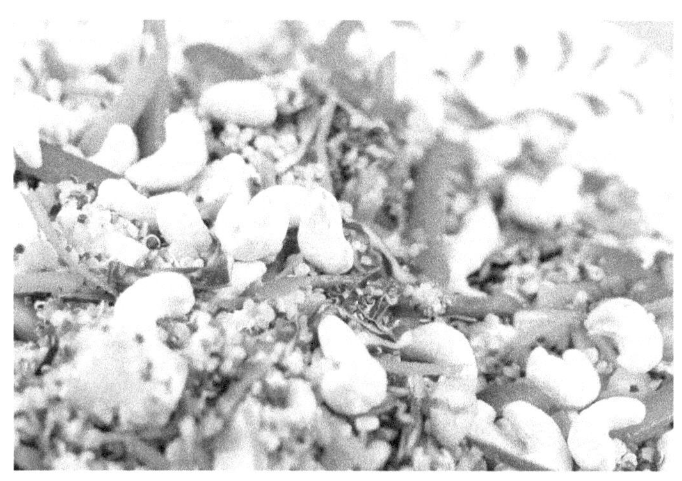

Vitamin C, which is vital for reproduction, is abundant in bell peppers. They also include a good amount of fiber, which helps control blood sugar levels and ward off cravings. Quinoa has all nine of the essential amino acids, making it a complete protein. In addition, it is a good source of zinc, iron, and magnesium—all of which are critical for healthy reproduction.

This meal is a tasty and wholesome way to get your recommended daily intake of quinoa and bell peppers. After the quinoa is cooked with garlic, onions, and spices, it is filled inside bell peppers that have been cut in half. After that, the peppers are roasted until soft.

Ingredients:

- 1 cup rinsed quinoa
- 1 chopped onion
- 2 minced garlic cloves
- 1 teaspoon cumin
- Half a teaspoon chili powder
- ¼ teaspoon salt
- ¼ teaspoon black pepper
- ¼ cup chopped fresh parsley
- ¼ cup vegetable broth or water

Guidelines:

- Set oven temperature to 375 F, or 190 C.

- Prepare the quinoa in a medium saucepan as directed on the package.

- In a large skillet over medium heat, warm the olive oil while the quinoa cooks. Add the onion and simmer for about 5 minutes, or until softened. Cook the garlic for a further 30 seconds after adding it.

Add the chili powder, cumin, pepper, and salt. Add another minute of cooking.

- Add the water or vegetable broth, quinoa, and parsley. After bringing to a boil, lower the heat, and simmer the quinoa for five minutes, or until it is soft.

- Stuffed bell pepper halves with the quinoa mixture.

- After placing the bell peppers in a baking tray, bake them for 20 minutes, or until they become soft.

Tips:

- You can roast the bell peppers before stuffing them for a more savory dish. In addition, you can add diced tomatoes, corn or zucchini to the quinoa mixture. You can use water in place of vegetable broth if you don't have any.

Benefits:

- Complete protein source
- High in fiber and vitamin C
- Good source of iron, magnesium, and zinc

Savor this recipe for Quinoa-Stuffed Bell Peppers as part of a nutritious and well-balanced diet to increase fertility.

CHAPTER 2

Green Goddess Goodness

2.1 Recipe 3: Spinach and Kale Power Salad

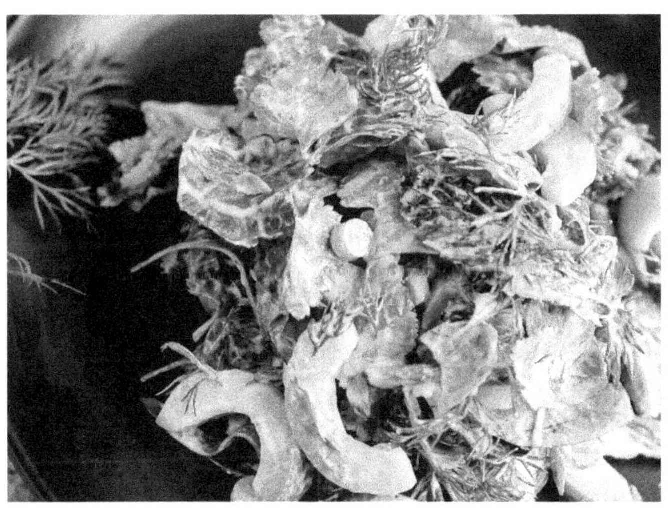

Vitamin C, iron, and folate are just a few of the minerals this salad is loaded with—all of which are critical for fertility. Additionally, it has a lot of fiber, which helps control blood sugar levels and ward off cravings.

Ingredients:

- 2 cups of Fresh spinach
- 1 cup of fresh kale
- ½ chopped strawberries
- ¼ chopped walnuts
- ¼crumbled feta cheese
- 2 tablespoons olive oil
- 1 teaspoon of balsamic vinegar
- 1 teaspoon of honey
- ½ teaspoon salt
- ¼ teaspoon if black pepper

These are the ingredients and quantities that this recipe calls for.

Guidelines

- Combine the spinach, kale, feta cheese, walnuts, and strawberries in a big bowl.

- Combine the olive oil, honey, balsamic vinegar, salt, and pepper in a small bowl.

3. Drizzle salad with dressing and toss to coat.
4. Present right away.

Tips:
- Add grilled chicken or prawns to make a salad higher in protein. Leave out the feta cheese to make the salad vegan. You may keep this salad in the fridge for up to two days.

Benefits:

- Rich in iron, which is necessary for supplying oxygen to the body's cells;

- High in vitamin C, which aids in shielding cells from harm.

- Rich in antioxidants, which help shield the body from damaging free radicals;

- High in folate, which is necessary to avoid neural tube problems.

Savor this flavorful and nourishing spinach and kale power salad as part of a nutritious diet to increase fertility.

2.2 Recipe 4: Broccoli and Avocado Smoothie

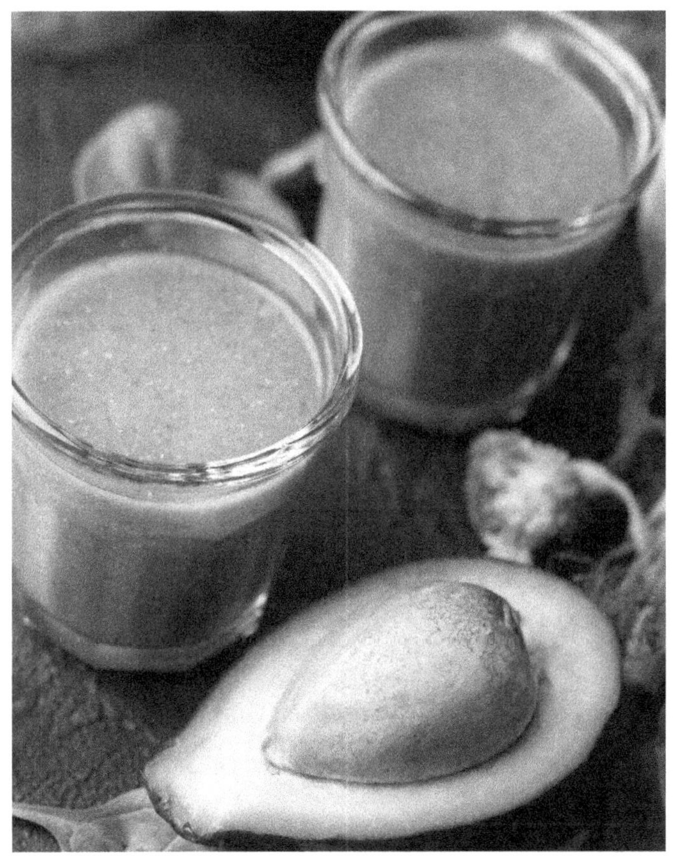

This smoothie is loaded with fiber, healthy fats, vitamin K, and C, all of which are critical for fertility. Additionally, it has a lot of protein, which helps maintain a feeling of fullness and satisfaction.

Ingredients :

- 1 Frozen broccoli florets
- ½ Avocado, peeled and pitted
- 1 of Banana, peeled and frozen
- 1 teaspoon of honey
- 1 cup of almond milk
- 1 cup of Spinach

Guidelines

- Fill a blender with all the ingredients, and process until smooth.

- Serve immediately.

Tips:

- Add additional frozen spinach or broccoli for a thicker smoothie.

- Add extra honey to make the smoothie sweeter.

- You may freeze this smoothie for up to two months.

Benefits:

- Rich in fiber, which can help control blood sugar levels and stave off cravings

- High in vitamin C, which aids in cell protection

- Good source of vitamin K, which is crucial for blood clotting. Healthy fats are necessary for the manufacturing of hormones.

- A good source of protein can assist maintain a feeling of fullness and satisfaction.

Additional Benefits of avocado and broccoli for fertility

- Broccoli is a cruciferous vegetable that contains sulforaphane, a compound that has been shown to protect sperm from damage.

- Avocados are a good source of monounsaturated fats, which can help to improve insulin sensitivity and ovulation.

Savor this tasty and nourishing smoothie made with broccoli and avocado as part of a balanced, healthful diet to increase fertility.

More recipes for smoothies to increase fertility:

- Berry Blast Smoothie: Blend together 1 cup mixed berries, 1/2 banana, 1/2 cup spinach, 1 cup almond milk, and 1 tablespoon honey.

- Mango Tango Smoothie: Blend together 1 cup frozen mango chunks, 1/2 banana, 1/2 cup spinach, 1 cup almond milk, and 1 tablespoon honey.

- Green Goddess Smoothie: Blend together 1 cup spinach, 1/2 banana, 1/2 avocado, 1 cup almond milk, and 1 tablespoon honey.

- Verdant Goddess Drink: Mix one cup spinach, half an avocado, half a banana, one cup almond milk, and one tablespoon honey in a blender.

Please be aware that there are numerous other tasty and nourishing smoothies you can have to increase your fertility; these are just a few examples. To discover your favorites, use your imagination and try a variety of fruits, vegetables, and protein sources.

CHAPTER 3

Protein Powerhouses

3.1 Recipe 5: Lentil and Sweet Potato Curry

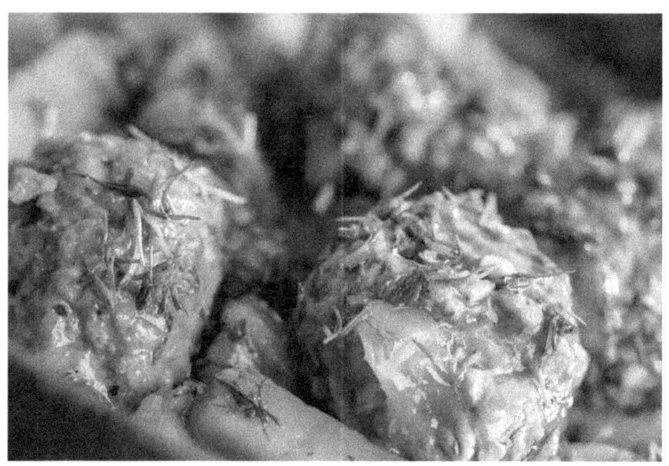

Protein, fiber, iron, and folate are just a few of the elements that are abundant in this substantial and tasty curry that are crucial for fertility. Antioxidants, which can help shield your cells from harm, are also abundant in it.

Ingredients:

- 1 chopped Onion
- 2 Garlic cloves, minced
- 1 tablespoon of Olive oil
- 1 tablespoon of Ginger Root, grated
- 2 tablespoons of Curry powder
- 1 teaspoon of Turmeric powder
- 1 teaspoon of Garam masala
- 1 large of Sweet potato, peeled and diced
- 1 cup of Red lentils
- 4 cups of Vegetable broth
- 1 Coconut milk   (13.5 ounces)
- Salt for teate
- Fresh cilantro, chopped for Garnishing.

Guidelines

- In a large pot over medium heat, warm the olive oil. Add the onion and simmer for about 5 minutes, or until softened.

- Include the curry powder, turmeric powder, ginger root, garlic, and garam masala. Cook, stirring regularly, for a further minute.

- Include the vegetable broth, sweet potatoes, and lentils. Once the lentils are soft, bring to a boil, then lower the heat and simmer for 20 minutes.

- Stir in salt and coconut milk. Cook for an additional five minutes.

- Add some fresh cilantro as a garnish and serve over quinoa or rice.

Tips:

- Add extra curry powder or a little teaspoon of cayenne pepper for a hotter curry.

- You can use water or ordinary milk in place of coconut milk. You may keep this curry in the fridge for up to three days.

Benefits:

- High in protein, which is essential for building and repairing tissues.

- Good source of fiber, which can help to regulate your blood sugar levels and prevent cravings.

- High in folate, which is essential for preventing neural tube defects.

- Contains antioxidants, which help to protect cells from damage.

- Rich in iron, which is important for carrying oxygen to the body's cells.

Additional advantages of sweet potatoes and lentils for fertility:

- Lentils are a good source of iron, which is important for ovulation.

- Sweet potatoes are a good source of beta-carotene, which is converted to vitamin A in the body. Vitamin A is essential for healthy reproductive organs.

Additional curry recipes to boost fertility:

- Chickpea and Butternut Squash Curry: Blend together 1 can (14 ounces) chickpeas, 1 cup butternut squash, 1 onion, 2 cloves garlic, 1 tablespoon ginger root, 2 tablespoons curry powder, 1 teaspoon turmeric powder, 1 teaspoon garam masala, 1 can (13.5 ounces) coconut milk, and salt to taste. Serve over rice or quinoa.

- Vegetable Curry: Blend together 1 cup mixed vegetables (carrots, zucchini, broccoli), 1 onion, 2 cloves garlic, 1 tablespoon ginger root, 2 tablespoons curry powder, 1 teaspoon turmeric powder, 1 teaspoon garam masala, 1 can (13.5 ounces) coconut milk, and salt to taste. Serve over rice or quinoa.

Tofu and Spinach Curry: Blend together 1 block (14 ounces) firm tofu, 1 cup spinach, 1 onion, 2 cloves garlic, 1 tablespoon ginger root, 2 tablespoons curry powder, 1 teaspoon turmeric powder, 1 teaspoon garam masala, 1 can (13.5 ounces) coconut milk, and salt to taste. Serve over rice or quinoa.

Please keep in mind that there are plenty other tasty and nourishing curries you may eat to increase your fertility; these are just a few examples. To discover your favorites, try experimenting with various veggies, proteins, and seasonings using your imagination.

3.2 Recipe 6: Grilled Salmon with Citrus Marinade

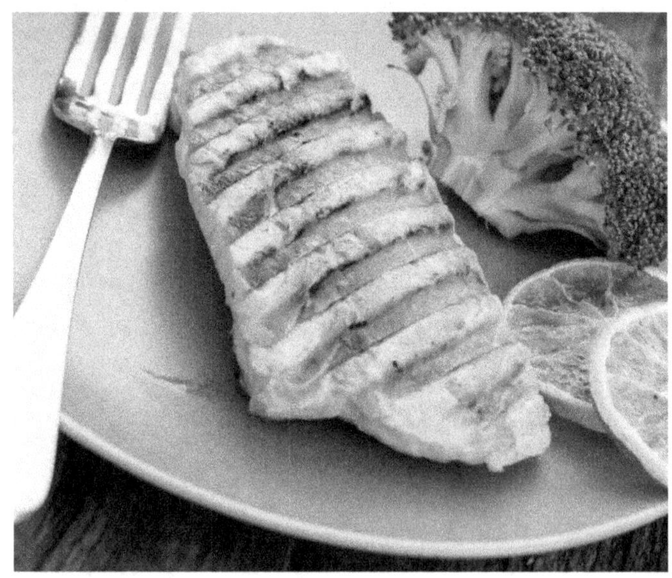

This citrus marinated grilled salmon recipe is a tasty and nourishing method to increase fertility. Omega-3 fatty acids, which are critical for the health of the reproductive system, are abundant in salmon. The fish is tenderized and given a zesty flavor by the citrus marinade.

Ingredients:

- 1 pound of cut-up salmon filets;
- ¼ cup of olive oil;
- ¼ cup of orange juice;
- ¼cup of lime juice;
- 1 tablespoon each of honey and soy sauce;
- ½ teaspoon of grated ginger;
- ½ teaspoon of salt;
- ¼ teaspoon of black pepper

Guidelines

- Combine the olive oil, soy sauce, ginger, orange and lime juices, honey, salt, and pepper in a big bowl.

- Coat the salmon filets by tossing them in the marinade.

- For at least thirty minutes and up to four hours, cover and refrigerate.

- Turn the grill's heat up to medium-high.

- Cook salmon filets on the grill for 4–5 minutes on each side, or until done.

Tips:

- Grill salmon filets over cedar planks for a smokier flavor.

- If you don't have a grill, you can bake the salmon filets in a preheated oven at 400 degrees F (200 degrees C) for 12-15 minutes, or until cooked through.

- Serve a side salad or steaming veggies with the salmon filets.

Benefits:

- Rich in vitamin D, which is crucial for calcium absorption
- High in omega-3 fatty acids, which are vital for reproductive health
- Good source of protein, which is necessary for tissue growth and repair

Additional salmon fertility benefits:

- It has been demonstrated that omega-3 fatty acids increase sperm motility and quality.

- A rich source of selenium, an antioxidant that may help shield cells from harm, is salmon.

- Choline, a vitamin crucial for brain development, is another component that can be found in abundance in salmon.

Delectable and nourishing Grilled Salmon with Citrus Marinade can be enjoyed as a part of a healthy, well-balanced diet to increase fertility.

More grilled fish recipes to increase ovulation

- Mango salsa and grill-tuned tuna: Cook tuna steaks on the grill for 4–5 minutes on each side, or until done. Accompany with chopped mango, red onion, cilantro, and lime juice for the mango salsa.

- Grilled Swordfish paired with Basil and Lemon Butter: Swordfish steaks should be cooked through after grilling for 4–5 minutes on each side. Accompany with melted butter, lemon juice, and chopped basil for the lemon-basil butter.

- Roasted asparagus with grilled halibut: Halibut filets should be cooked thoroughly after grilling for 4–5 minutes on each side. Serve over roasted asparagus that has been seasoned with salt, pepper, and olive oil.

CHAPTER 4

Fertility-Boosting Fruits

4.1 Recipes 7: Berry Blast Smoothie Bowl

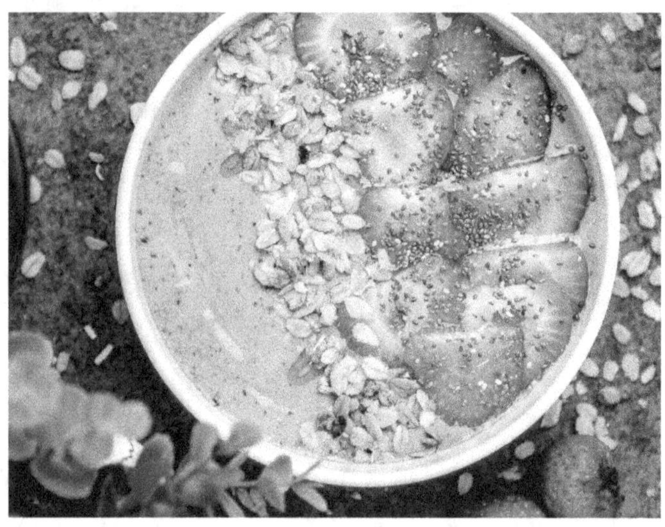

Indulge in a delightful and nutrient-dense breakfast with this vibrant Berry Blast Smoothie Bowl, specially crafted to support fertility. Packed with an array of berries, pomegranate, and wholesome ingredients, this smoothie bowl is a powerhouse of antioxidants, vitamins, and fiber, essential for optimal reproductive health.

Ingredients:

1. 1 cup mixed berries (blueberries, raspberries, and strawberries)
2. 1/4 cup pomegranate arils
3. 1/4 cup plain Greek yogurt
4. 1 tablespoon chia seeds
5. 1 tablespoon flax seeds
6. 1 tablespoon hemp seeds
7. 1/2 cup almond milk
8. 1 tablespoon honey
9. 1/4 teaspoon vanilla extract
10. Additional toppings of your choice (granola, nuts, berries, or pomegranate arils)

With this vivid Berry Blast Smoothie Bowl, you can embrace a morning habit that promotes your reproductive quest while also nourishing your body. This delicious concoction is a symphony of nutrients and flavors that supports reproductive health as well as general well-being.

- A Profusion of Berries

The stars of this smoothie bowl, the berries, are not only tasty but also a powerhouse of vital elements that support fertility. Antioxidants, found in abundance in strawberries, raspberries, and blueberries, shield cells from harm and support a healthy reproductive system.

- Power of Pomegranates

The bowl's ruby-like gems, the pomegranate arils, add a plethora of antioxidants along with a rush of flavor. Pomegranate juice is a great compliment to a diet that increases fertility because studies have proven it to enhance sperm quality and motility.

- Flax, Hemp, and Chia Seeds: A Triple Threat of Beneficiary

Nutritious powerhouses, chia, flax, and hemp seeds are abundant in omega-3 fatty acids, which are critical for reproductive health. Blood sugar regulation, hormone production, and general reproductive health are all aided by omega-3 fatty acids.

- Greek Yogurt: A Base Packed with Protein

In addition to adding a creamy texture to the smoothie bowl, plain Greek yogurt has a substantial amount of protein, which is essential for the development and repair of tissues during pregnancy. Probiotics, or good bacteria, are another ingredient in Greek yogurt that promote intestinal health and general wellbeing.

- Honey: A Hint of Sugarcosiness

The natural sweetener honey gives the smoothie bowl a little sweetness without lowering its nutritional content. Honey has been demonstrated to have anti-inflammatory qualities and is an antioxidant source.

- A Plant-Based Alternative for Almond Milk

A creamy and smooth base for the smoothie bowl is provided by almond milk, a dairy-free substitute. Vitamin E, an antioxidant that promotes reproductive health, is abundant in it.

- Vanilla Extract: A Tasty Complement

The flavor of the smoothie bowl is enhanced by vanilla essence, a delicate yet fragrant component that doesn't overpower the flavors of the yogurt and berries.

- Extra Garnishes: A Custom Touch

You can top the smoothie bowl with granola, almonds, pomegranate seeds, or berries to personalize it and improve its nutritious value. Berries give more antioxidants and vitamins, nuts supply healthy fats and protein, and granola adds more crunch and fiber.

- Delight in a Healthful Morning Routine

This nutrient-dense, flavor-packed Berry Blast Smoothie Bowl is a great way to start the day because it will fuel your body and aid in your fertility journey. You will be enjoying a symphony of flavors and nutrients with each mouthful, supporting optimal reproductive health and general well-being.

4.2 Recipe 8: Tropical Fruit Salad with Honey-Lime Dressing

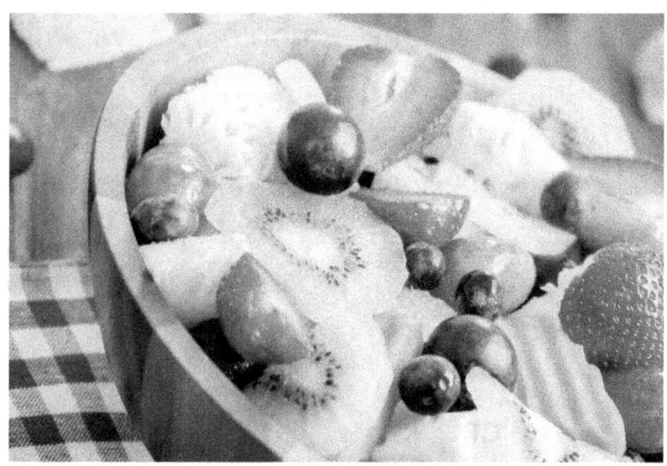

Take your taste buds on a tropical culinary journey with this colorful Tropical Fruit Salad with Honey-Lime Dressing. It's a lovely blend of exotic fruits and a spicy dressing that promotes fertility and general well-being.

Ingredients:

- 1 cup mixed tropical fruits (mango, pineapple, papaya, guava)
- ½ cup strawberries, halved
- ¼ cup blueberries
- 1 tablespoon honey
- 1 tablespoon lime juice
- ¼ teaspoon vanilla extract

Additional toppings of your choice (mint leaves, chopped nuts, pomegranate arils)

Guidelines:

- Place blueberries, strawberries, and assorted tropical fruits in a big bowl.

- Combine the honey, lime juice, and vanilla extract in a small bowl.

- Drizzle the fruit salad with the honey-lime dressing, gently tossing to coat.

- For cold flavors, refrigerate for a minimum of half an hour.

- Garnish with extra toppings of your choosing and serve cold.

A Harmonious Mix of Tropical Berries

- Mango, pineapple, papaya, and guava, the stars of this fruit salad, are not just delicious but also packed with essential nutrients for fertility. Mangoes are rich in vitamin C, which supports embryo development. Pineapples contain bromelain, an enzyme that has been shown to improve uterine health. Papayas are a good source of vitamin A, essential for healthy reproductive organs. Guavas are packed with antioxidants, which protect cells from damage and promote overall well-being.

A Spicy Lime-Honey Dressing

- The dressing's base ingredients, lime juice and honey, provide a lovely harmony of acidity and sweetness that accentuates the tastes of the tropical fruits. Honey adds a hint of sweetness to the salad without lowering its nutritional content. In addition to adding a zesty flavor, lime juice is high in vitamin C, which is crucial for fertility.

A Reviving and Healthful Delight

- This delightful and nourishing Tropical Fruit Salad with Honey-Lime Dressing nourishes your body and aids in your reproductive quest. You'll be enjoying a symphony of tropical flavors and vital nutrients with every meal, supporting optimal reproductive health and general well-being.

CHAPTER 5

Vital Veggies

5.1 Recipe 9: Roasted Carrot and Ginger

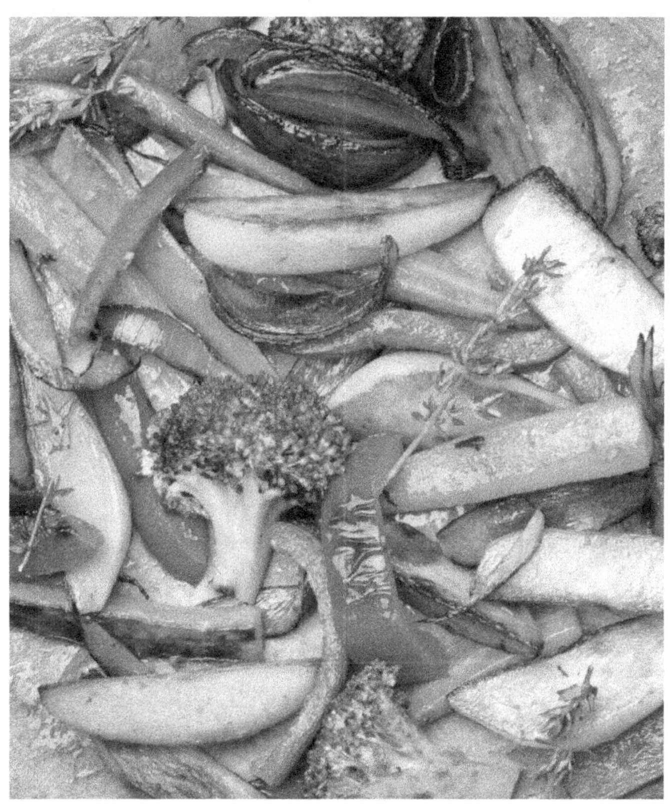

This Roasted Carrot and Ginger Soup is a gourmet concoction that will nourish your body and assist your fertility journey. Soak in its warmth and comforting flavors. Packed with vital nutrients, antioxidants, and anti-inflammatory chemicals, this silky smooth soup supports the best possible reproductive health and general well-being.

Ingredients:

- 2 pounds carrots, peeled and chopped
- 1 tablespoon olive oil
- 1 tablespoon ground ginger
- ½ teaspoon salt
- ¼ teaspoon black pepper
- 4 cups vegetable broth
- ¼ cup coconut milk (optional)

Additional toppings of your choice (fresh cilantro, pumpkin seeds, chopped nuts, or a dollop of Greek yogurt)

Guidelines:

- Set oven temperature to 400 F, or 200 C.
- Arrange carrots in a chopped state on a baking sheet and lightly coat with olive oil.
- Season the carrots with salt, pepper, and ground ginger.
- Roast the carrots for thirty to forty minutes, or until they are soft and caramelized.
- Heat the veggie broth in a big pot over medium heat.
- Include the roasted carrots and heat through.
- Simmer for 10 to 15 minutes on low heat.
- Puree the soup with an immersion blender or a standard blender until it's creamy and smooth.
- To add even more richness, stir in coconut milk, if using.
- Use your taste buds to adjust the seasonings.

- Garnish with extra toppings of your choosing and serve warm.

A Harmony of Tastes and Elements

- The main ingredient in this soup, carrots, are not only delicious but also a great source of important nutrients that promote fertility. They contain a lot of beta-carotene, which the body uses to make vitamin A. For the development of embryos and healthy reproductive organs, vitamin A is necessary.

- The spicy and delicious ginger gives the soup a cozy, energizing feel. Strong anti-inflammatory properties have been demonstrated, along with enhanced uterine blood flow and support for regular menstrual cycles.

- An optional addition that adds a hint of creaminess and is a great source of good fats is coconut milk. Lauric acid, which has antiviral and antibacterial properties and helps maintain a healthy immune system, is also abundant in it.

A Comforting and Filling Hug

This warming and reassuring soup of roasted carrots and ginger will nourish your body and aid in your fertility journey. You'll be enjoying a symphony of flavors and vital nutrients with every spoonful, supporting optimal reproductive health and general well-being.

5.2 Recipe 10: Asparagus and Mushroom Stir-Fry

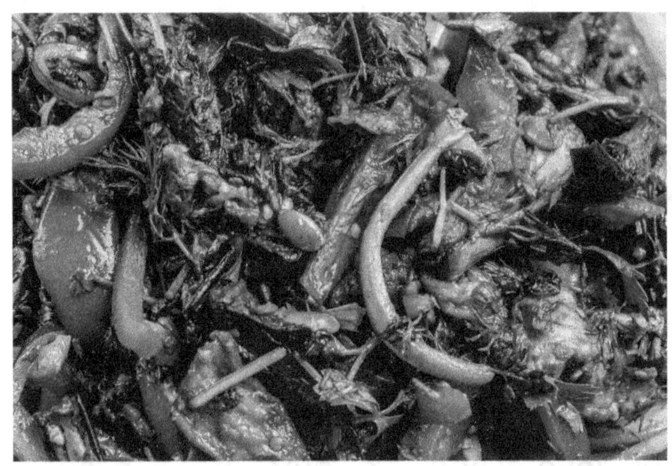

Take your taste buds on a gastronomic journey with this colorful stir-fried asparagus and mushrooms. It's a delicious blend of crunchy asparagus, earthy mushrooms, and a rich sauce that promotes fertility and general health.

Ingredients:

- 1 bunch of asparagus, trimmed and cut into 2-inch pieces
- ½ pound sliced mushrooms (cremini, shiitake, or a combination)
- 1 tablespoon olive oil
- 1 tablespoon minced garlic
- 1 tablespoon grated ginger
- 2 tablespoons soy sauce
- 1 tablespoon honey
- 1 tablespoon rice vinegar
- ¼ teaspoon sesame oil
- Additional toppings of your choice (sesame seeds, chopped nuts, or a dollop of Greek yogurt)

Guidelines:

- In a large skillet or wok, heat the olive oil over medium-high heat.
- Add the asparagus and mushrooms, and stir-fry for 5 to 7 minutes, or until the mushrooms

are browned and the asparagus is crisp-tender.

- Combine the grated ginger, soy sauce, honey, rice vinegar, and sesame oil in a small bowl.
- Drizzle the stir-fried asparagus and mushrooms with the sauce, then gently toss to cover.
- Cook for a further two to three minutes, or until the sauce has somewhat thickened.
- Garnish with extra toppings of your choosing and serve warm.

A Concerto of Fertility-Inducing Components

- The main ingredient in this stir-fry, asparagus, is not only delicious but also a great source of important nutrients for fertility. Folic acid, which is necessary to avoid neural tube abnormalities, is abundant in this food. In addition, vitamin C, an antioxidant that shields cells from harm, is present in asparagus.

- The earthy companions to asparagus, mushrooms offer a variety of nutrients along with umami flavor. They provide an excellent supply of copper, which is necessary for the development of embryos. Antioxidants, which shield cells from harm and enhance general wellbeing, are also found in mushrooms.

- The sauce, a flavorful concoction of soy sauce, honey, rice vinegar, and sesame oil, adds extra nutrients and a symphony of flavors. B vitamins, which support hormone production, are found in soy sauce. Honey adds a hint of sweetness to the stir-fry without lowering its nutritional content. In addition to providing a tart flavor, rice vinegar is a wonderful source of antioxidants. The savory flavors are accentuated by sesame oil, which also includes vitamin E, an antioxidant that promotes reproductive health.

A Nutritious and Flavorful Delight

- This tasty and nourishing stir-fried dish of asparagus and mushrooms will fuel your body and aid in your fertility journey. You'll be enjoying a mix of flavors and vital nutrients with each bite, supporting optimal reproductive health and general well-being.

Conclusion

As you embark on your fertility journey, incorporating fertility-enhancing foods into your diet is a crucial step towards achieving optimal reproductive health. By embracing a nutrient-rich diet, you provide your body with the essential building blocks to support healthy ovulation, sperm production, and embryo development.

Here are some key tips for incorporating fertility-enhancing foods into your diet:

1. Prioritize Whole Foods: Focus on consuming whole, unprocessed foods that retain their natural nutrients. These include fruits, vegetables, whole grains, legumes, nuts, seeds, and lean protein sources.

2. Embrace Variety: Aim for a diverse range of colors and textures on your

plate. Each food offers a unique blend of nutrients, so a varied diet ensures you're getting a comprehensive range of essential vitamins, minerals, and antioxidants.

3. Include Fertility-Boosting Foods: Incorporate specific foods known to support fertility, such as leafy green vegetables, fatty fish, berries, and nuts. These foods provide nutrients like folate, omega-3 fatty acids, antioxidants, and vitamin E, which play crucial roles in reproductive health.

4. Limit Processed Foods: Reduce your intake of processed foods, sugary drinks, and excessive caffeine. These items can contribute to inflammation and nutritional imbalances, potentially hindering fertility.

5. Cook with Healthy Fats: Incorporate healthy fats into your cooking, such as olive oil, avocado oil, and nut butters.

These fats support hormone production and nutrient absorption.

6. Plan and Prepare: Plan your meals and snacks ahead of time to make healthy choices more convenient. Prepare batches of whole grains, fruits, and vegetables to have on hand for quick and nutritious meals.

7. Seek Guidance: Consult a registered dietitian or nutritionist for personalized advice on incorporating fertility-enhancing foods into your diet. They can help you create a meal plan tailored to your individual needs and preferences.

8. Mindful Eating: Practice mindful eating, paying attention to your hunger cues and enjoying your food without distractions. This helps you make conscious food choices and avoid overeating.

9. Stay Hydrated: Drink plenty of water throughout the day to stay hydrated and support overall health. Water is essential for nutrient transport and waste removal, both crucial for fertility.

10. Consistency is Key: Make gradual and sustainable changes to your diet rather than drastic overhauls. Consistency is key to reaping the long-term benefits of a fertility-enhancing diet.

Remember, incorporating fertility-enhancing foods into your diet is just one aspect of a holistic approach to optimizing reproductive health. Regular exercise, stress management, and adequate sleep are also essential for overall well-being and fertility. By nurturing your body and mind, you create a supportive environment for a successful fertility journey.